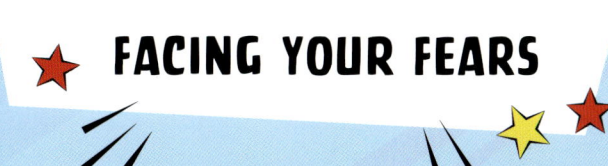

**FACING YOUR FEARS**

AF208399

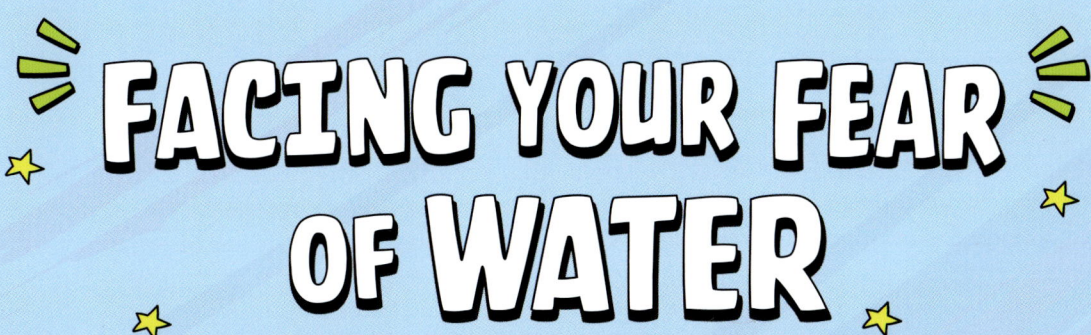

# FACING YOUR FEAR OF WATER

BY HEATHER E. SCHWARTZ

Consultant:
Tawnya M. Ward, PsyD, LP
Clinical Psychologist
Shakopee, Minnesota

PEBBLE
a capstone imprint

Published by Pebble, an imprint of Capstone.
1710 Roe Crest Drive, North Mankato, Minnesota 56003
capstonepub.com

Library of Congress Cataloging-in-Publication Data is available on the Library of Congress website.
ISBN: 9781666355543 (hardcover)
ISBN: 9781666355604 (paperback)
ISBN: 9781666355666 (ebook PDF)

Summary: Explores the reasons why many people are afraid of water and provides simple tips for facing this fear safely.

Editorial Credits
Editor: Christopher Harbo; Designers: Sarah Bennett and Jenny Bergstrom; Media Researcher: Julie De Adder; Production Specialist: Katy LaVigne

Image Credits
Getty Images: Daniel Grill, 19, Destinations by DES–Desislava Panteva Photography, 8, FatCamera, 9, 14, kali9, 5, 17, Marilyn Nieves, cover, 13, Ruslan Dashinsky, 18; Shutterstock: All For You, 20 (twig), Anton Starikov, 20 (bowl), Domira (background), cover and throughout, FamVeld, 11, iuliia_n, 21, Kapitosh (cloud), cover and throughout, Lopolo, 15, Marina_ph, 4, Marish (brave girl), cover and throughout, Microgen, 12, New Africa, 20 (toys), Petr Bonek, 6, photka, 20 (rocks), Pongchart B, 7, wavebreakmedia, 10

Printed and bound in the USA. 4882

# TABLE OF CONTENTS

Words in **bold** are in the glossary.

# WATER WORRIES

Are you scared of the water? That feeling is telling you to be **cautious**. It's keeping you safe. But that doesn't mean you need to stay scared. If you do, you'll miss out on all kinds of fun.

It's OK if you're fearful. With a few simple steps, you can learn to love the water.

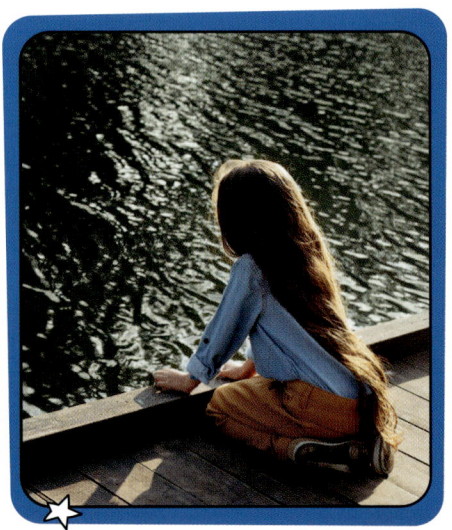

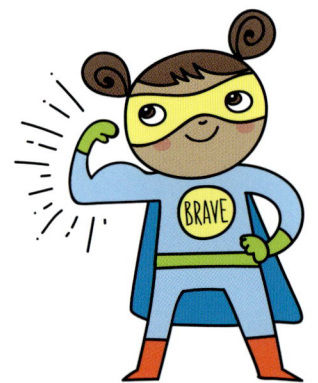

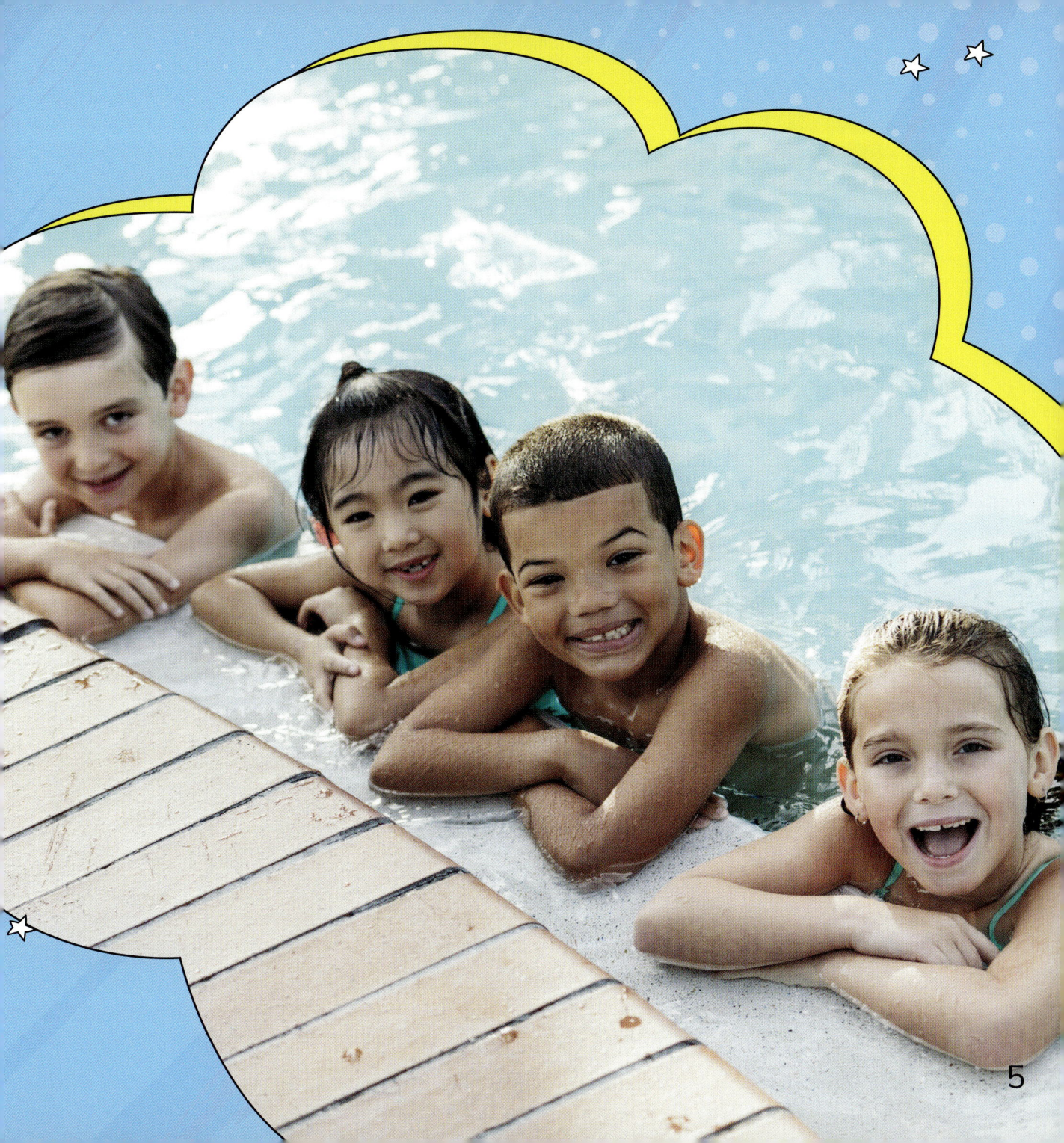

# START SMALL

Get used to the water by starting small. Dangle your feet in the pool. Stay on the steps. Wade into the lake only up to your knees.

Take it slow to get more comfortable. Are you afraid to get your face wet? Try kissing the water first. Then try blowing bubbles!

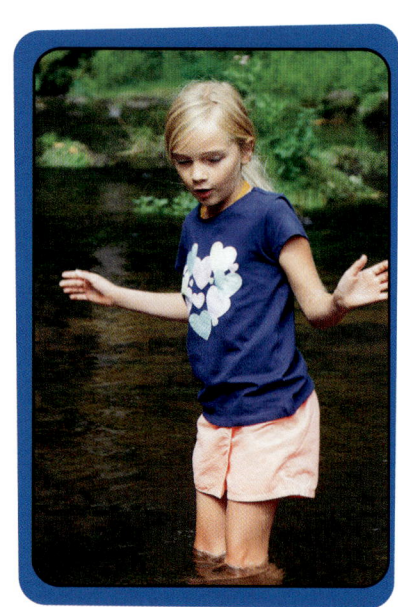

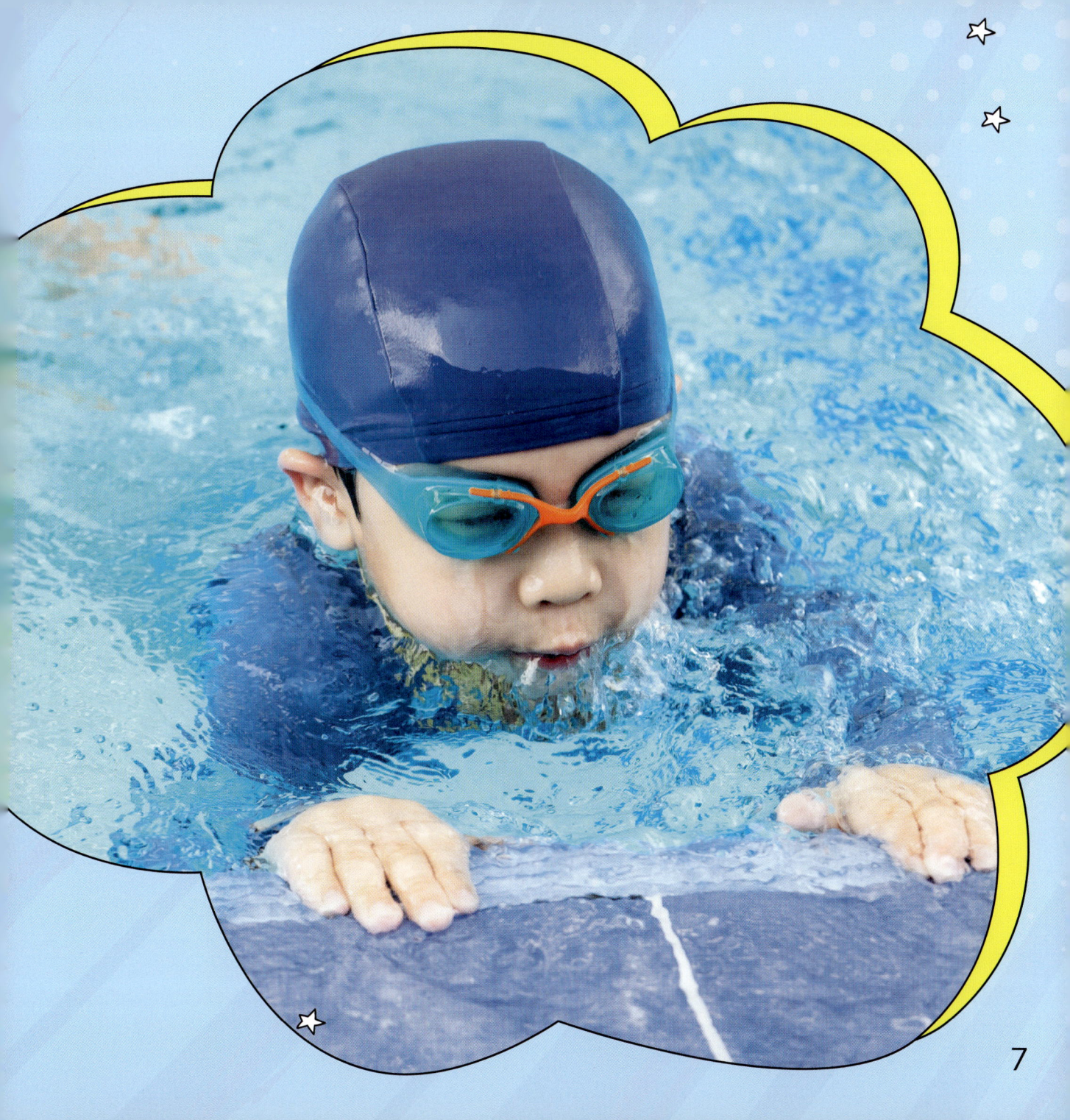

Swim gear can help you enjoy the water too. A nose clip keeps water out of your nose. Ear plugs keep water out of your ears. Goggles keep water out of your eyes.

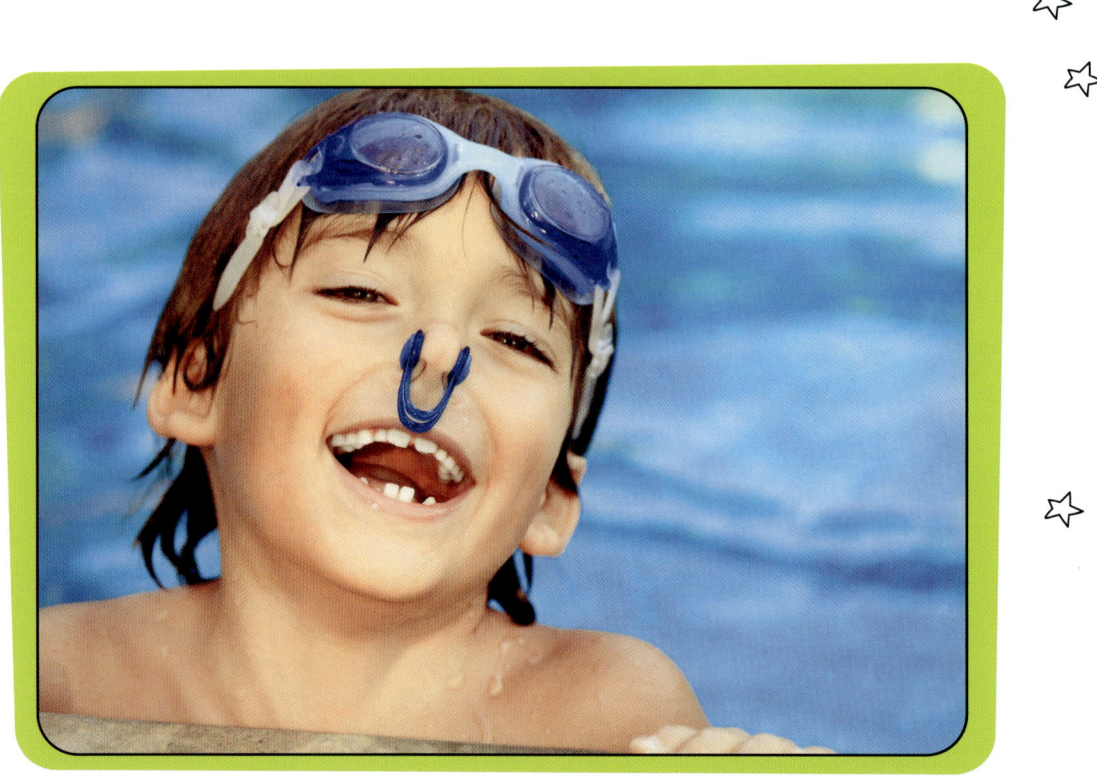

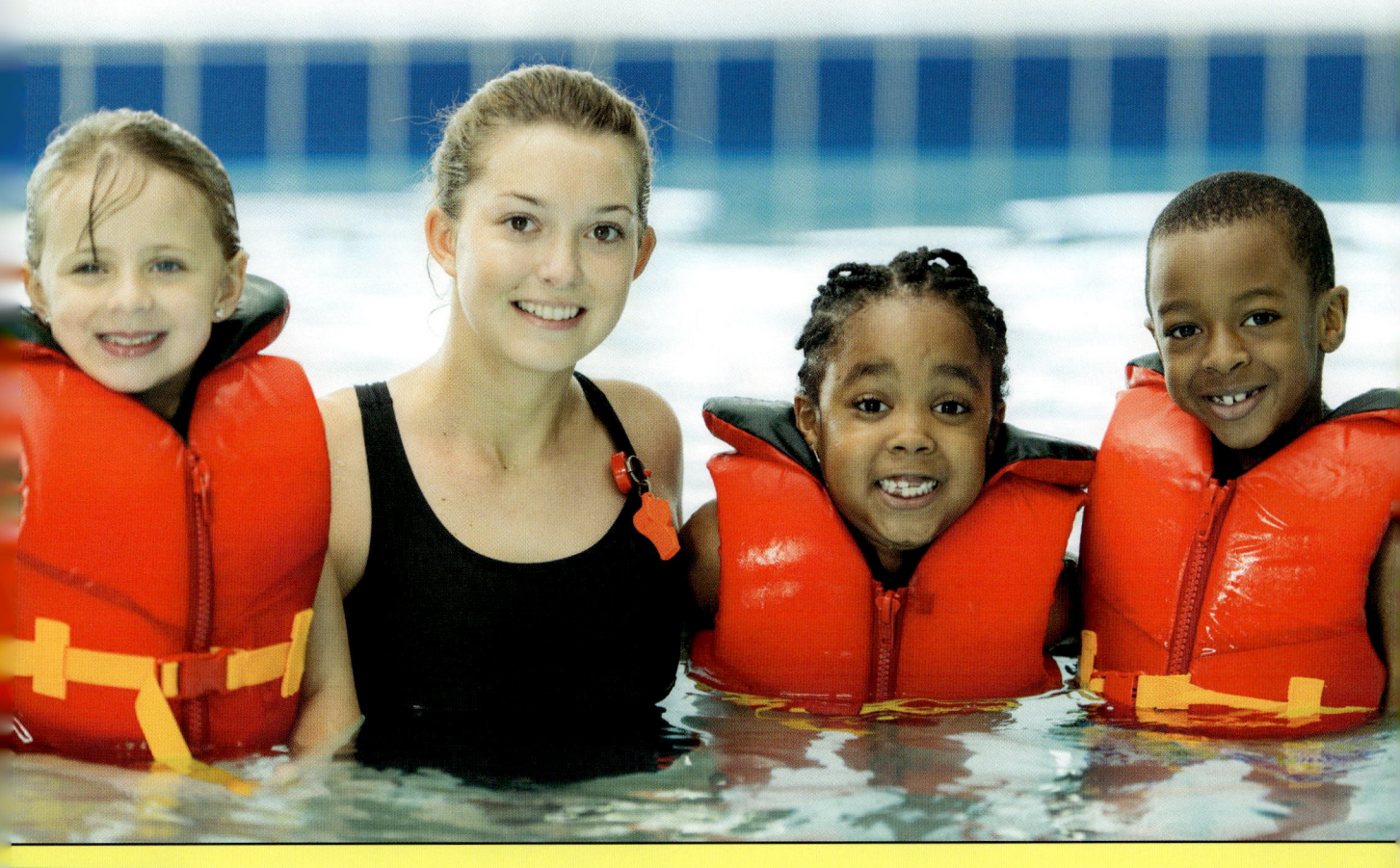

A **swim vest** is another idea. It will keep you from sinking. It can help you feel safe in the water.

# TAKE SWIMMING LESSONS

When you know how to swim, the water is not so scary. You could take swimming lessons. Or maybe a trusted adult could teach you.

Learning to swim is like learning to ride a bike. It takes time and **courage**. You have to try new things in the water. That might be scary. But it can also be fun.

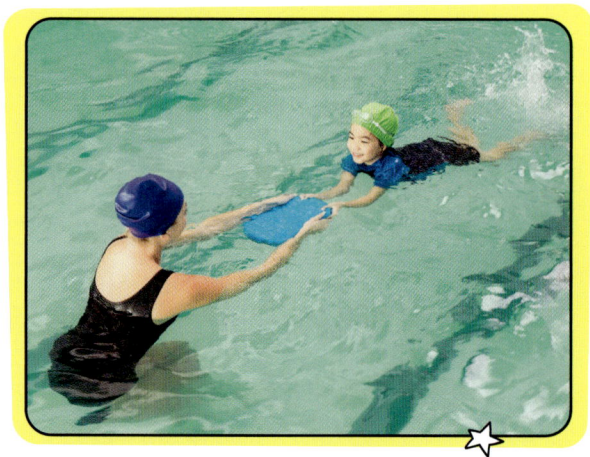

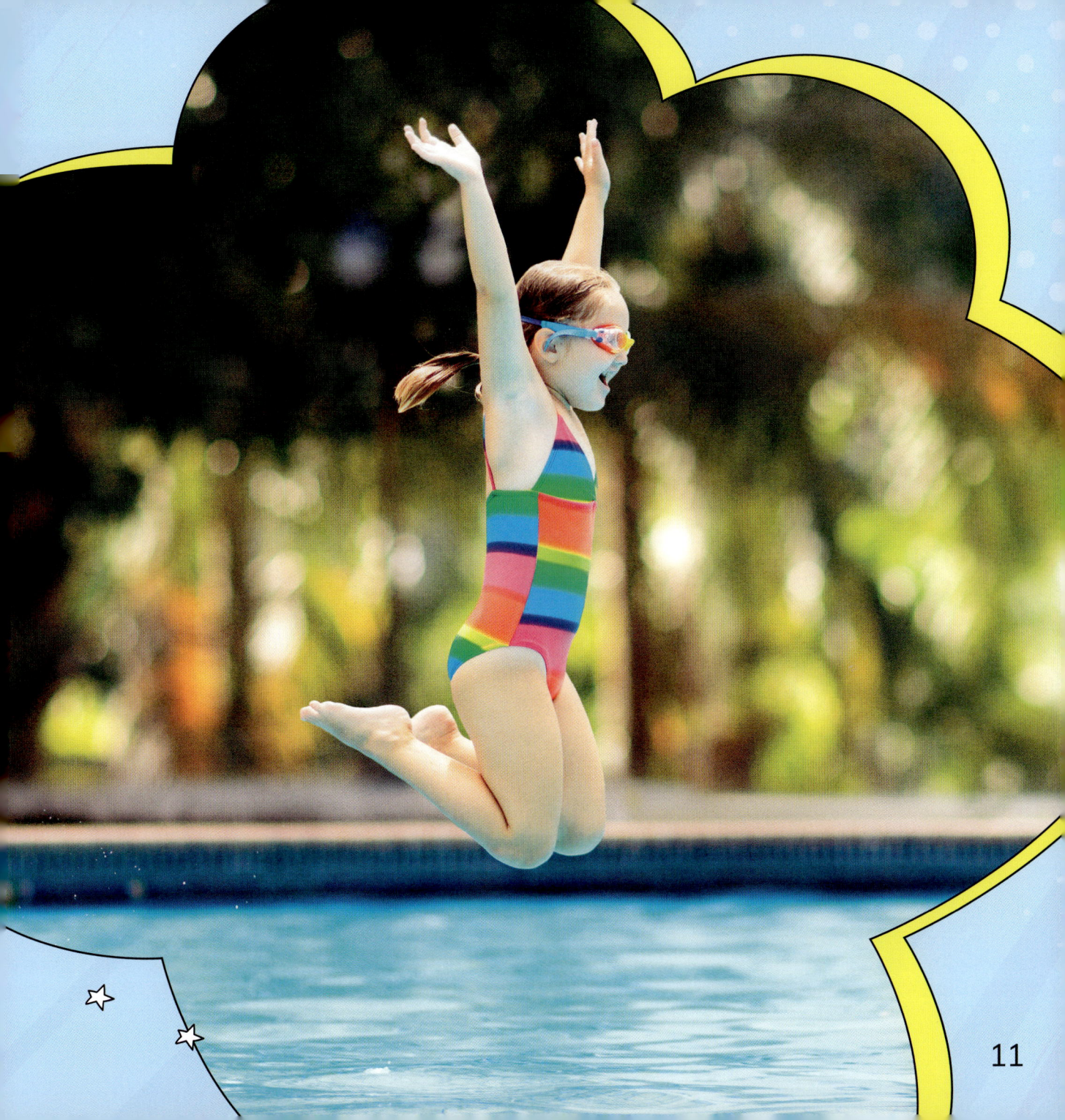

Swimmers have special **skills**. They know how to stay safe in the water. They learn to **tread** water. They learn to float on their backs. They learn how to hold their breath underwater. You can learn the same skills. You can be a swimmer too!

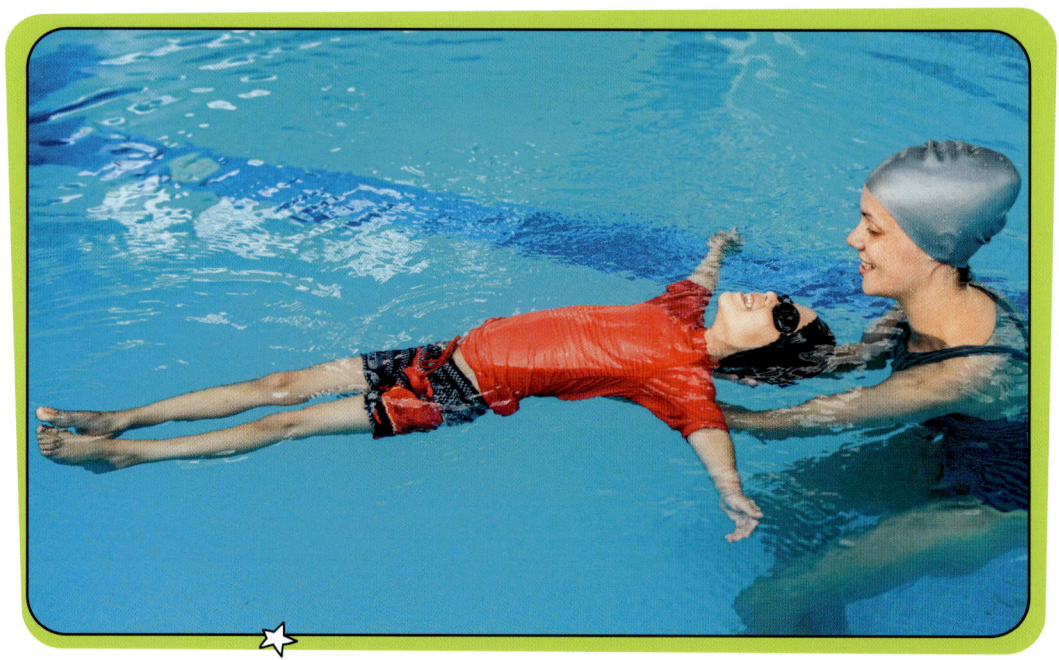

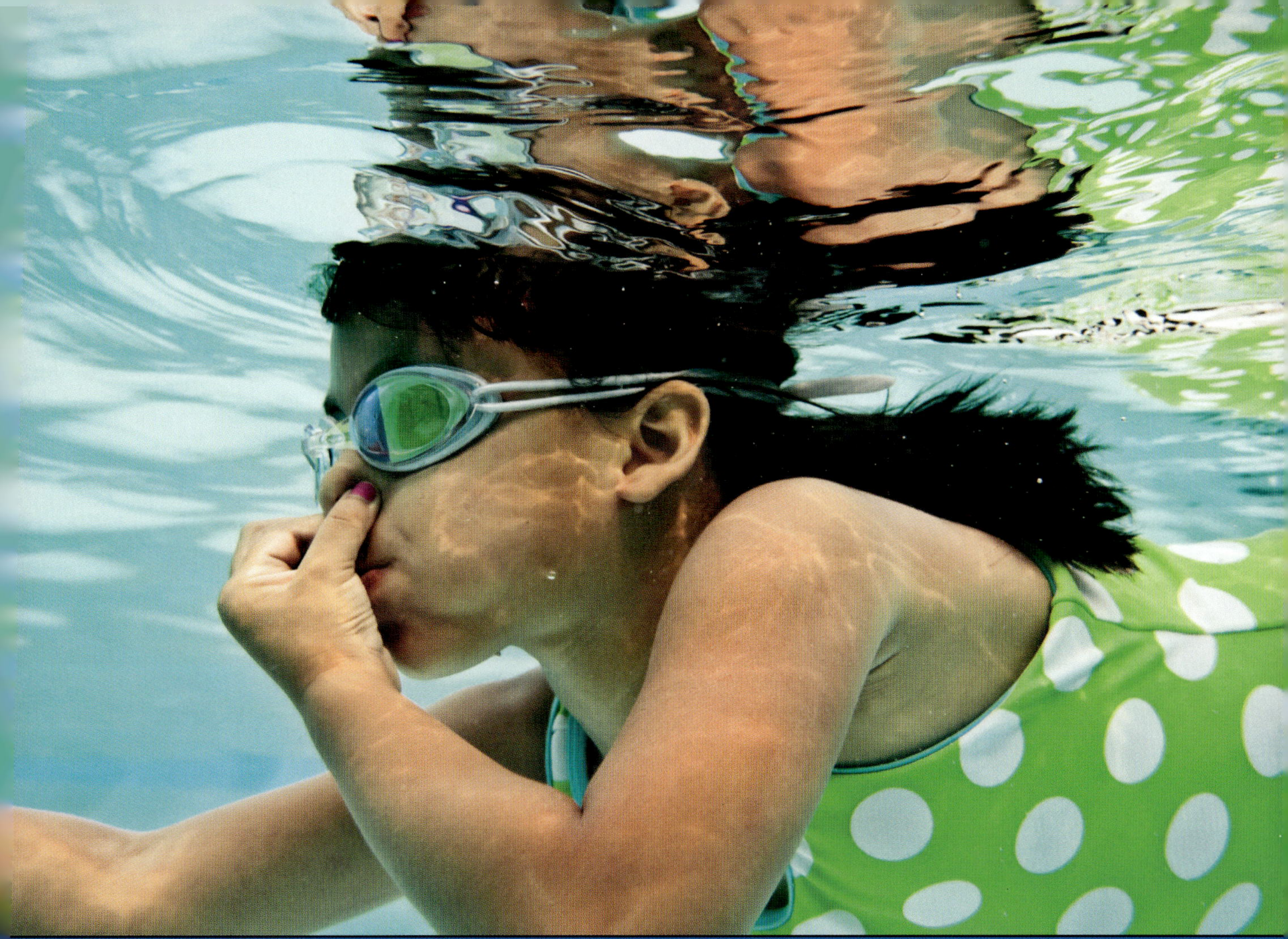

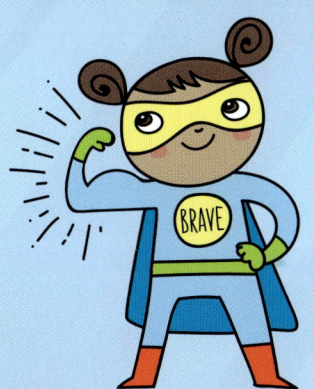

# PLAY IT SAFE

Following the rules around water can help you feel less fearful. You will know you are staying safe. Listen to adults. Be sure someone is watching you. That could be a trusted adult or a **lifeguard**.

Swimming and boating have different rules. You may not have to wear a **life jacket** while you swim. But you should always wear one on a boat.

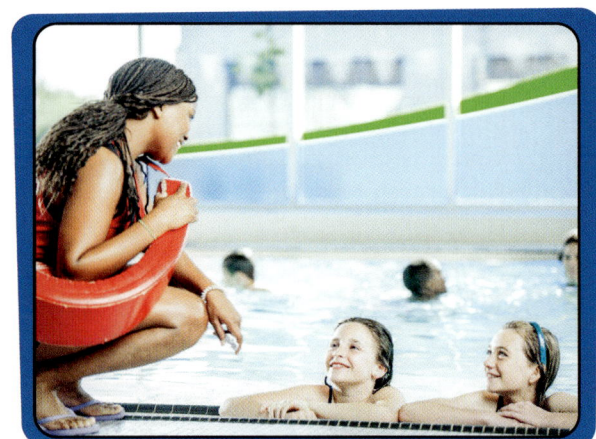

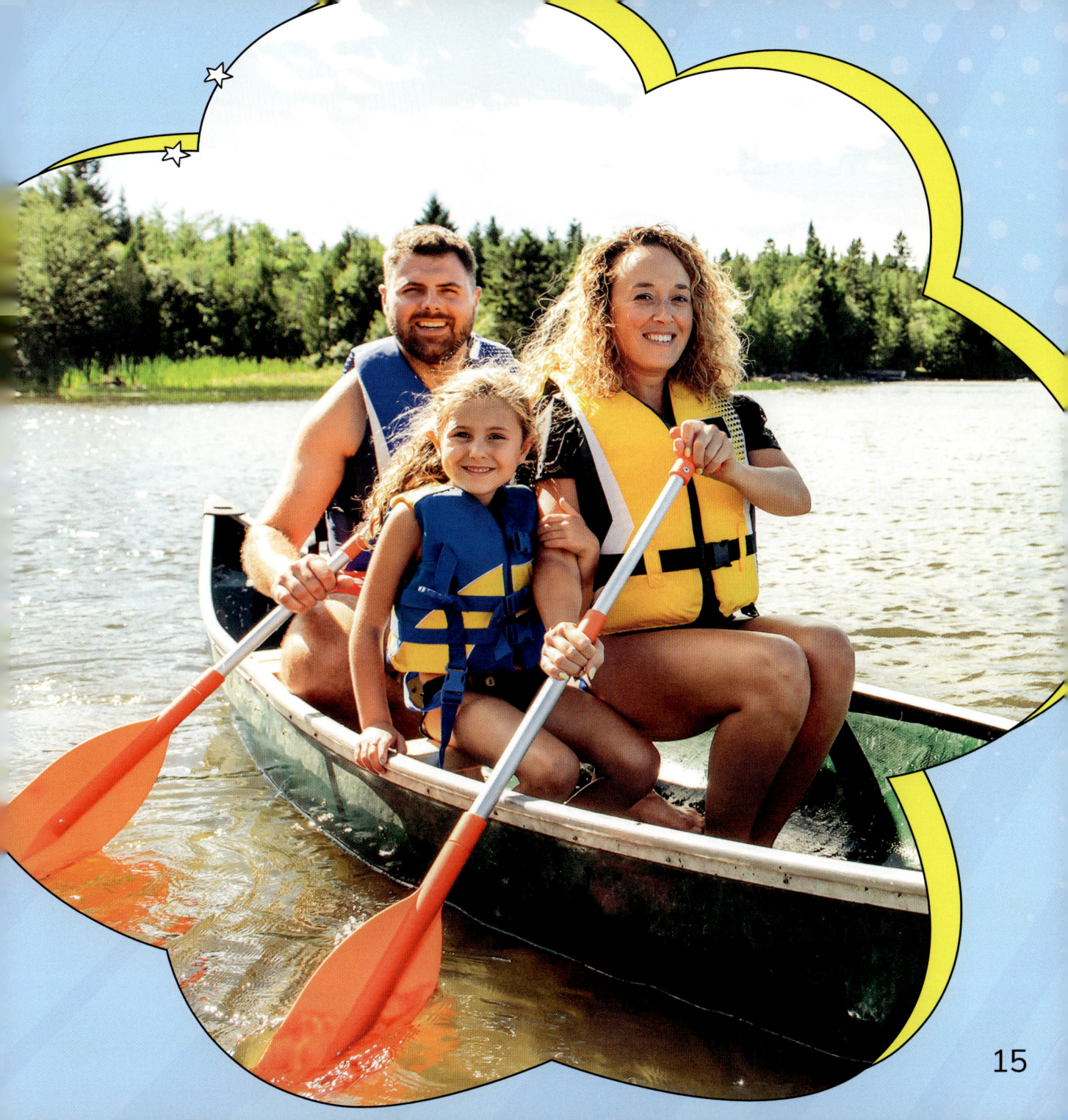

You can make your own rules to feel safer too. Afraid of the deep end? Decide to stay where you can touch the bottom. Scared of the diving board? Try the small slide instead. Don't worry about what your friends are doing. Go at your own **pace**.

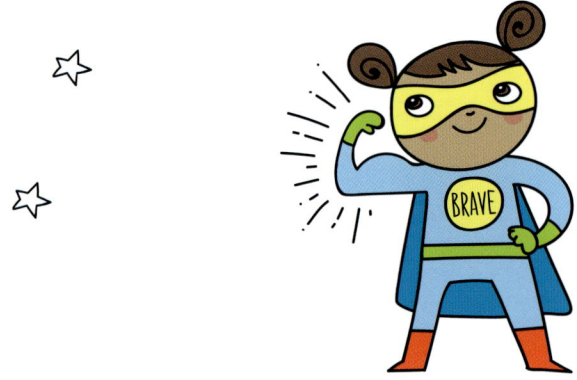

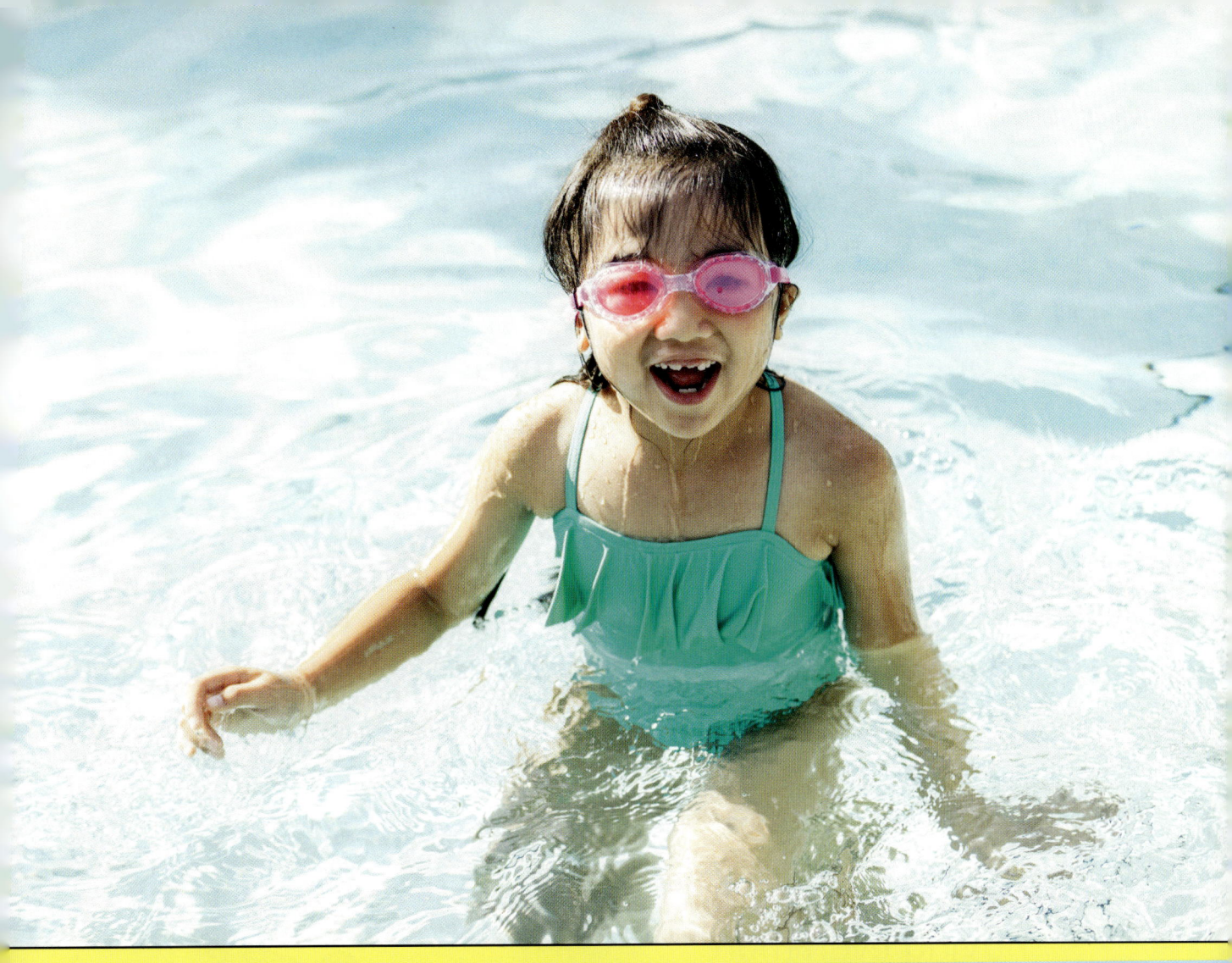

# WATER CAN BE WONDERFUL

Fear of the water is normal. But don't let it get in your way. Try water activities that feel safe. Skip the ones that scare you.

Keep building your swimming skills. You'll build your **bravery** at the same time. Soon, you'll be having even more fun in the water.

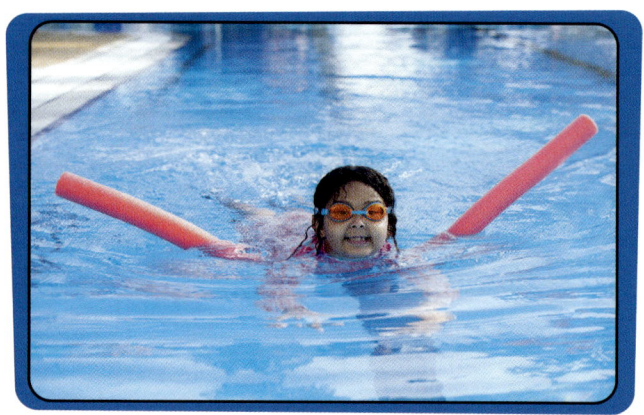

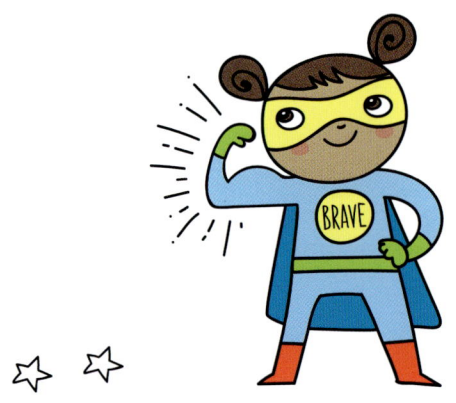

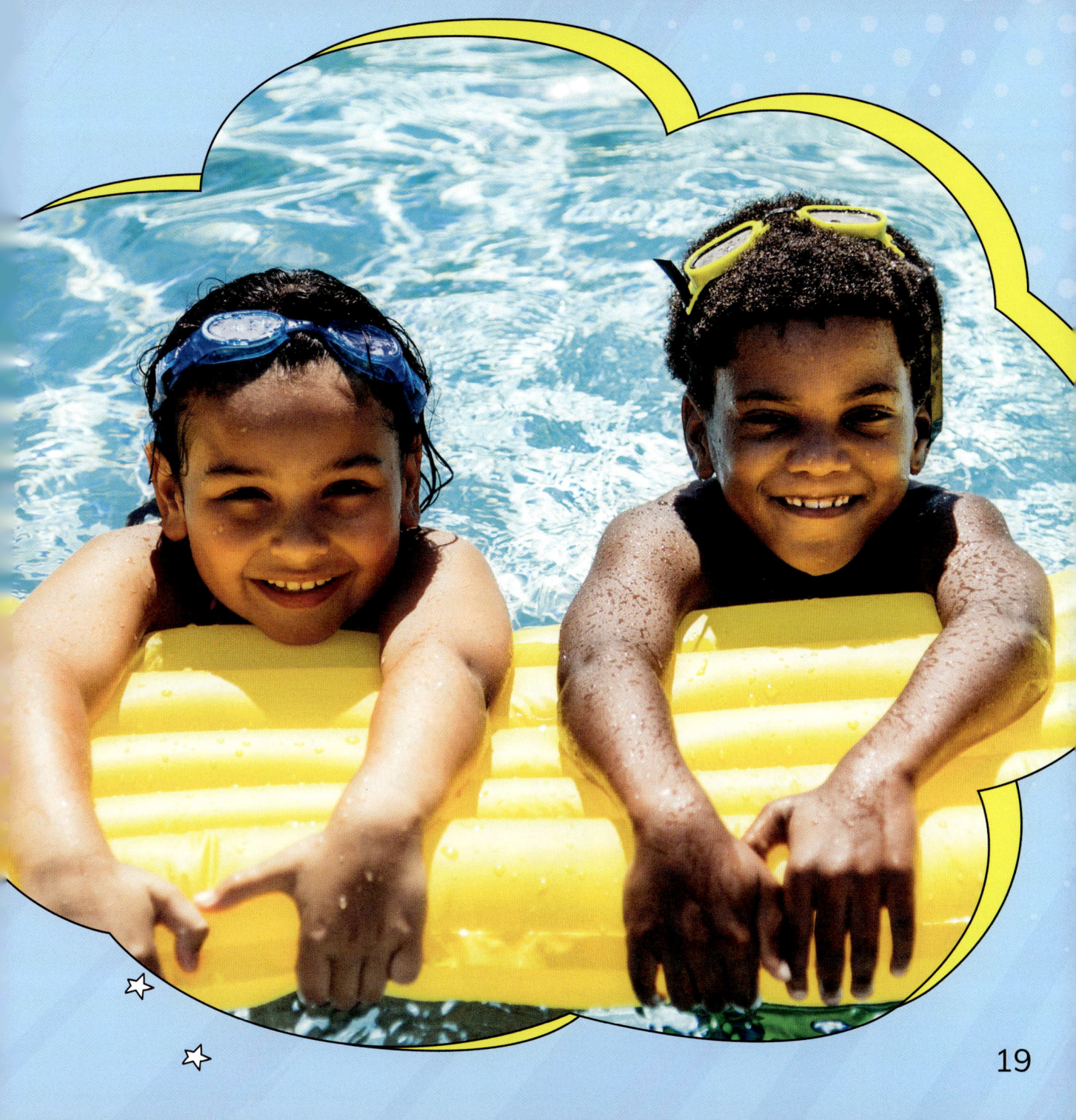

# SINK OR FLOAT

Life jackets are made of foam that floats. What other types of materials do you think would float? Test different items to find out which ones sink and which ones float.

## What You Need

- large mixing bowl
- water
- pencil
- paper
- small objects, such as toys, plastic cups, rocks, and sticks

## What You Do

1. Fill a large mixing bowl with water.

2. Draw two columns on a piece of paper. Label one column "sink" and the other one "float."

3. Pick one of your small objects and place it in the water. Watch to see if it sinks or floats.

4. Write the name of the object in the column that matches what happened.

5. Repeat steps 3 and 4 with the rest of your items.

6. Look at your two columns. How many objects sank? How many were able to float? Why do you think some floated and others sank?

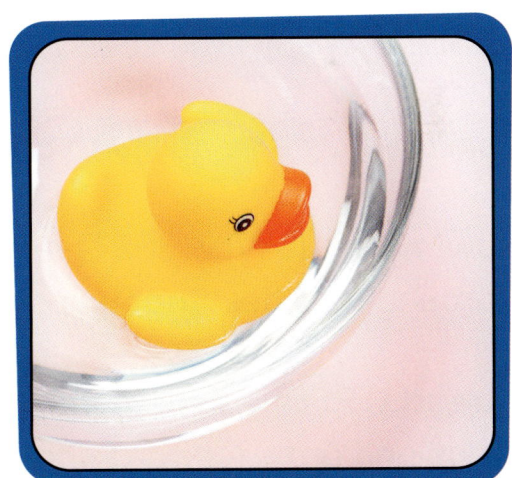

# GLOSSARY

**bravery** (BRAVE-ree)—having courage

**cautious** (KAW-shuhss)—careful about avoiding danger or risk

**courage** (KUHR-ij)—bravery in times of danger

**life jacket** (LIFE JAK-it)—a device to keep you afloat if you fall in the water

**lifeguard** (LIFE-gard)—a person trained to help swimmers

**pace** (PAYSS)—the speed at which something moves

**skill** (SKIL)—the ability to do something well

**swim vest** (SWIM VEST)—a thin flotation device worn around the chest that helps small children swim

**tread** (TRED)—to float upright in water by moving your legs and arms forward and backward

## READ MORE

Kesselring, Susan. *Around Water*. New York. AV2 by Weigl, 2020.

Bassier, Emma. *Water Safety*. Minneapolis: Pop!, 2021.

Francis, Trace Wilkins. *Safety First*. Deer Park, N.Y.: Annie Jean Publishing, 2020.

## INTERNET SITES

*American Red Cross: Water Safety for Kids*
redcross.org/get-help/how-to-prepare-for-emergencies/types-of-emergencies/water-safety/water-safety-for-kids.html

*Britannica Kids: Water*
kids.britannica.com/kids/article/water/390625

*National Geographic Kids: The Ocean's Weirdest Creatures!*
natgeokids.com/uk/discover/animals/sea-life/strange-sea-creatures

# INDEX

# ABOUT THE AUTHOR

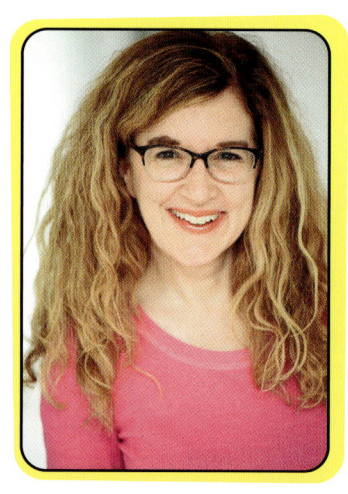

photo by Dan Doyle

Heather E. Schwartz has written hundreds of children's books. Her favorite way to swim is floating on her back. She lives in upstate New York with her husband, two kids, and two cats named Stampy and Squid.